the
TEX-MEX DIET!

Be a Trophy in 30 days to weight loss
and have a jovial attitude to go with it!

PEACHES MONROE

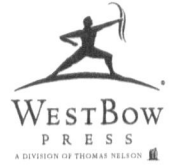

WestBow
PRESS
A DIVISION OF THOMAS NELSON

WestBow Press books may be ordered through booksellers or by contacting:

WestBow Press
A Division of Thomas Nelson
1663 Liberty Drive
Bloomington, IN 47403
www.westbowpress.com
1-(866) 928-1240

Because of the dynamic nature of the Internet, any web addresses or links contained in this book may have changed since publication and may no longer be valid. The views expressed in this work are solely those of the author and do not necessarily reflect the views of the publisher, and the publisher hereby disclaims any responsibility for them.

Any people depicted in stock imagery provided by Thinkstock are models, and such images are being used for illustrative purposes only.

Certain stock imagery © Thinkstock.

ISBN: 978-1-4497-8466-9 (sc)
ISBN: 978-1-4497-8465-2 (e)
ISBN: 978-1-4497-8467-6 (hc)

Library of Congress Control Number: 2013902440

Printed in the United States of America

WestBow Press rev. date: 2/11/2013

A Word from the Author

If you are currently or have been in the past an over-eater, this book is for you! But first, promise me something. I want you to promise me that after reading this book in its entirety and consulting with your physician, you will give it 31 days. That's all. Just 31 days to the rest of your life. Overeating is a habit which slaves its victims. It can harm your health. After reading this book, you will eat your way into losing weight. So many diet plans ask you to starve or limit your food intake in such a way that success cannot be achieved over the long haul. With our plan, you will eat regular food and lose weight.

When you're overweight, people can be very cruel and tactless. They make comments that are very hurtful. Have you ever experienced this? I have; and, it hurts. As a woman, I have had to face a lot of confrontations. However, I am very grateful for all of my problems. I became stronger as I conquered each obstacle. I lived above my problems and circumstances.

At the start of my effort to overcome my overweight problems, I had to develop a positive mental attitude about it. When you feel that you can overcome any problem, you're taking into account that you do not have to do it entirely on your own. You have extra help and strength that God gives. My mother would always tell me to call on Jesus when trouble times hit. I did a lot of calling. Through it all, I realized that He is the supernatural help that I needed on a daily basis. Look up Jeremiah 33:3 in the Bible. It says, "Call unto me, and I will answer thee, and shew thee great and mighty things, which thou knowest not". If you feel weak, or perhaps your problems or circumstances seem too much for you, just call upon Him and He will answer you. He will show you a way out of your difficulties. James 1:5 says, "If any of you lack wisdom, let him ask of God, that giveth to all men liberally, and upbraideth not; an it shall be given him". He will guide you and direct you in overcoming any problem. Try Him. May God Bless You!

The key to my success was to realize the source of my weight problems. I found the source to be overeating and/or gluttony.

I have taken numerous nutritional courses and have consulted with dietitians as appropriate in publishing this book.

When and Why I Overeat

One of the main reasons I used to overeat was my family. They constantly reminded me of the things I shouldn't have eaten. They watched me religiously and criticized me if I ate something they felt I shouldn't have eaten. They told me they did this because I needed them to. They called it "helping me out". My solution to their method was to eat whatever I wanted before they arrived home from work or school. Does this sound familiar to you?

The second reason I used to overeat was because I was lonely. Being overweight can be very lonely at times. Food becomes your best friend. Being lonesome caused me to seek intimacy through food. Of course, after I stuffed myself with all the empty calorie foods, I was still lonely and depressed. The more I ate, the more I became unhappy. Have you ever experienced this?

I found that my top seven reasons why I indulged in food was:

1. *Stress*
2. *Loneliness*
3. *Worry*
4. *Fear*
5. *Tension*
6. *Anxiety*
7. *Loss of something, such as a relationship or self-worth.*

Why do you overeat?

1.
2.
3.
4.
5.
6.
7.

Whatever your reasons for overeating, YOU ARE NOT ALONE. I have been there. We've all been there.

Promise me you will do the next three things:

1. *Believe in yourself*
2. *Be patient*
3. *Record everything in your memoirs.*

~NO PROBLEM IS too DIFFICULT to SOLVE~

Thirty-one Day Program Introduction

Don't you just love how the Southern cooks prepare food? Don't you just love to eat Mexican food? Well, if you answered yes to either question or you're been deprived of this fine cooking, this is the book for you.

Tex-Mex is a type of foodstuff primarily found in the state of Texas. It is basically American food with a Mexican flair to it. Oftentimes, Tex-Mex meals have more meat than beans. However, beans can be substituted for meat. When you get started, my only warning is that you take it slowly. Tex-Mex foods are usually spicy and have a hotness you may not be accustomed to. Nevertheless, you will build up tolerance, and you'll have the best time dieting and losing weight.

Before you get started with any health-changing program and/or weight-loss regime, please consult your family physician about it. Take this book to your physician and have him or her take a look at our weight-loss program and make the appropriate recommendations.

I love the cooking from Texas, Mississippi, Louisiana, and Alabama. I also love Mexican food. So I came up with a plan where I could have both and still lost weight. Wow,

I had the best of both worlds. I must be honest though. I still sometimes felt intimidated when I saw individuals who were fit. I could feel myself become a little envious or spiteful. But, a little voice inside would whisper to me, *"It's not their fault you let yourself go. They probably don't order fast foods. They probably don't snack and eat at all times of the day. And, they probably don't think of food as being their friend."* Sometimes, I would hate to hear that voice. I realized it was imperative that I change my way of thinking. So-, I did. After designing a plan that incorporated all the foods I love, I worked the plan, and lost weight. I lost a lot of it. You will too.

The obesity rate in the United States is staggering. According to the Health and Human Services and the Center of Disease Control Prevention (CDC), as of January 2012, the most recent national data on obesity prevalence among U.S. adults, adolescents, and children show that more than one-third of adults and almost 17% of children and adolescents were obese in 2009–2010. Differences in prevalence between men and women diminished between 1999–2000 and 2009–2010, with the prevalence of obesity among men reaching the same level as that among women.

Age differences in obesity prevalence varied between men and women. The prevalence of obesity was higher among older women compared with younger women, but there was no difference by age in obesity prevalence among men. Among children and adolescents, the prevalence of obesity was higher among adolescents than among preschool-aged children.

Obesity: Body mass index (BMI) was calculated as weight in kilograms divided by height in meters squared and rounded to one decimal place. Obesity in adults was defined as BMI greater than or equal to 30. BMI calculates "fatness" based on someone's height and weight (CDC, 2012).

Table. Obesity cut points for adults 5'4" and 5'9" in height

Height	Obesity weight range
5'4"/1.63 meters	174 pounds or more/79 kilograms or more
5'9"/1.75 meters	203 pounds or more/92 kilograms or more

This constitutes there are at least 20 million individuals in the United States have diseases, such as, cancer, diabetes, heart disease, high cholesterol, kidney, and other medical issues that could be related to weight. Today, over 60 percent of us in the United States have a higher body mass index (BMI) higher than medically recommended.

I disagree when others say, "Diets don't work." They do work – temporarily, if you're disciplined. In my opinion, the problem is that, some of us, like me, are not disciplined over a long period of time. Listen, diets are man-made. We weren't born to diet. Diets made me focus on food and not on my emotions, which was causing me to overeat. On this regimen, you will eat regular foods.

I have tried so many diets and I have had success in a few, temporarily at least. But, the weight would always come back. Where was my discipline? I finally found the answer to losing weight and keeping it off. It's eating. Yes, the best way to diet is to eat! I ate the foods I love. That's it. It is that simple.

It's also about your attitude. I have learned that if you're encouraging and positive, you will lose weight. I know, I know, I get it. It sounds crazy but it works. I will show you how in this book. This technique will enhance your entire life. You will finally be able to address those hurts that are causing your weight problems. Are you ready?

Before you begin, please get a medical checkup with your physician. Make sure you have your physician's approval to go on this thirty-one day regimen. Keep a record of the foods you eat on a daily basis and you will have optimal success.

Part One:

This day is the best day of the rest of your life. You will lose weight feel better. The first step is to imagine how you will look at your goal weight, dress size, or waist size. Snatch that vision from your mind and believe it. Do you believe you can reach your goal weight? If the answer is yes, you're ready. If not, just give this book away or put it in a safe place until you are ready.

Okay, are you ready? Great, let's do this.

Keys to Success:

1. You are approved! You will lose weight.
2. Focus on your strengths and confront your weaknesses.
3. Trust yourself and believe you can lose the weight.
4. If you believe you can lose the weight, you will.
5. Stay encouraged and positive, you will lose weight.

On this thirty-one day regimen, you will not have to weight yourself. You will try on a garment that is your goal to wear. My goal garment was a size 4 - lined linen skirt. I tried it on at least a hundred times during my thirty one days. Each time before I tried it on, I said to myself, "Today is the day, I will wear this skirt". I must have made that statement at least 120 times. But – one day I *did* wear it. What I had been saying actually came true.

For the next thirty-one days, you will feel better physically, eat great foods by eating more, learn to love yourself, and discover how to maintain wonderful, loving, friendships, and relationships.

Diets that have excessive fat content have been associated with acute medical conditions like obesity, heart disease, diabetes, and cancer. Health officials stress the significance of lowering of fat intake to no more than 30% of total calories consumed, which comes out to be around 58 grams of fat per day. There are ways a person can reduce their fat intake. One way is by reducing whole fat dairy products, beef, pork, and cream based sauces. In the process of doing this, an individual should be careful not to lower the omega 3 fatty acids consumption. Scientific research state that omega 3 fatty acids help prevents a large range of medical problems like heart disease, arthritis, and depression. Dietary sources of omega 3 fatty acids include flaxseeds, walnuts, hemp seeds, soybeans, and dark green leafy vegetables.

When pursuing weight lost, avoid all fried foods or food stuff cooked in oils. Try to cook vegetables and meats in vegetable broth than butter or margarine. Pay close attention to the serving size and the number of servings per package. Try to eat more bean dishes and or soy than red meat. Choose leaner cuts of red meat and try to cut fat that's seen. When cooking chicken, remove the skin after cooking it. This will keep the meat tender. Finally, increase the consumption of fruits, vegetables, and whole grains rather than snacks high in calories and fat. When preparing green garden salads, try to keep the salad dressing to a minimum by having them on the side of the salad and not on top of the salad.

The TexMex Diet stresses the importance of whole grains, beans, fruits, and veggies. Raw nuts and seeds should be eaten in moderation. Fish such as salmon, tuna and the like are high in omega 3 fats and should be eaten at least once per week.

The TexMex Diet emphasizes following a low fat diet. A low fat diet is a diet that contains fewer than 30% or no more than 58 grams of fat per day. This type of diet plan is highly unlikely to result any harm to a healthy person. However, children require additional fat to maintain appropriate and normal growth and development and should not be restricted.

For more information about how to cut the fat out of your diet, check out the following web pages:

- The Low Fat Vegetarian Archive located at www. fatfree.com.
- The official web site of the American Dietetics Association located at www.eatright.org.

Part Two:

What is your body shape? Are you shaped like a pear, apple, straight, curvy, or athletic?

Here are a few descriptions.

Pear – individuals are usually smaller above the waist. They tend to pack weight onto their lower bodies, such as hips, thighs, and rear end.

Since the lower half of your body is more generous that the upper, the idea is to create some balance, by focusing the eye on the upper half, and drawing it away from the hips and thighs.

Tips for women include:

While this can be done in a number of ways, some wardrobe basics to keep in mind are as follows as appropriate:

1. Wear darker fabrics as lowers and bright, lighter tops
2. Choose flared skirts and dresses
3. Choose fabrics and fits that skim the hips, then fall straight
4. Shoes make a big difference - wearing heels will add length to your body.

Apple – individuals have a less defined waist than other figure types. They tend to carry their weight in the midsection.

Tips for women include:

1. Use clothes to accentuate your midriff, so it looks less like an apple and more like an apple core. At the same time, draw attention to your favourite bits - that cleavage, those legs, and anything else you really like.
2. Body control underwear will work wonders to define your middle area too, pulling you in at the waist.
3. Don't hide in baggy trousers. Show off your lovely legs with straight or boot-cut trousers. Look for flat-fronted trousers with a wide waistband to draw attention away from the stomach.
4. Open up the neckline. V-necks and scoop-necks are good for apple-shaped ladies as you often have a great bust. Don't be afraid to show it off.
5. Use structured tailored jackets to give definition to your upper body and show off good shoulders. Look for single-breasted versions with one or two buttons.
6. Wrap dresses are always a winner for an apple body shape as they fit nicely over a fuller bust. A side tie on the dress will draw attention away from the stomach.

Straight – individuals are usually stick-like straight and with few curves. They usually develop a potbelly when weight is gained.

Tips for women include:

1. Look for garments that will create volume, with details such as frills, fluted edges and ruffles.
2. Boot cut jeans are perfect for you - the slight flare is flattering, and the slim fit shows off a petite waist and great bum.
3. If you want to create the impression of bigger boobs, look for chunky statement necklaces that fall around the bust area.
4. Stay away from clothes with a large print, as they can drown out your dainty features.
5. Draping will give soft lines across the body and will create volume in your more petite areas.
6. Add a push-up
7. Trapeze-style jackets have lots of fabric to play with. Cinch it in at the waist with a belt: the material underneath will create a peplum effect, adding volume to the hips.

Curvy – individuals have breasts and hips that are larger in relation to their waist. Their weight gain is usually distributed to all parts of their body, though some seem to carry it in their hips and thighs.

Tips for women include:

1. Use large type-sleeves on a jacket to emphasise your shoulders.
2. An A-line skirt teamed with a fitted top will mirror your fabulous hourglass shape.

3. A short flared ruffle detail on a skirt creates a line down from the waistline to the hip, which will exaggerate your curvy hips.
4. You can wear any shape skirt, but the pencil skirt is the most flattering on you. Team with a simple shirt, tucked in and unbuttoned to reveal a little cleavage.
5. Straight-legged jeans that skim your thighs and are cropped at the ankle work well for you. Boot cut jeans will balance your curves - look for darker shades and ones with large pockets on the bum.
6. High-waisted, wide-legged trousers will emphasise the curve of your hip without making your bottom half look big.
7. Use draping to your advantage. Not only will it accentuate your curves - look for diagonal draping from the waist to hip area - but it will also disguise the tummy area.
8. Wear fitted clothes but make sure they're not too tight. Consider going one size up so your clothes really mirror your figure, rather than pull at it.

Athletic – individuals usually have broad shoulders and narrow hips. They usually carry extra weight in their midsection.

Tips for women include:

1. Short, fitted dresses show off your slender shape and long legs. Floppy dresses with simple spaghetti straps instantly add dimension and femininity.

2. Stay away from round or plunging necklines - they will make your breasts look smaller - and opt for an empire-line cut instead.

3. Your slim hips and long legs can accommodate the frilliest underwear, and you can add oomph to your cleavage with a padded bra.

4. Leggings look great as they show off your slim legs and allow you to wear something with more volume or detail on top. You can get away with skinny and straight-legged jeans too.

5. Use A-line skirts to add definition to your waist. You can experiment with lengths - show off those lovely legs. Flat waistbands on skirts will add some structure to your middle.

6. Look for feminine details in your clothes to soften any hard lines. Ruffles on tops will work wonders.

7. Pay attention to the fabrics of the clothes you buy - look for feminine prints and soft materials. Give the illusion of a waistline - pull it in with a waist-cinching belt.

Petite – individuals that are five foot three or under, and have a small frame, you've got the petite body figure.

Tips for women include:

1. You look great in well-tailored, form-fitting clothes (nothing baggy of course) and showing lots of leg will make you look taller. Invest in a tailored jacket to give structure to your shape.

2. Dresses are your friends - opt for ones in a single colour from shoulder to knee.

3. Research brands that specialise in petite sizes. Alternatively, get handy with a needle and thread and alter the length of garments yourself.
4. Draw attention to the top half of your body with stripes and patterns. Block colours on the bottom half will elongate your figure.
5. Avoid colours that are too 'girly' - sugary pinks, lilacs etc - as they can appear childlike.
6. Use large but delicate accessories to help draw attention to the top half of your body. Hooped earrings are ideal.
7. Consider the length of garments - opt for longer lines to make you look taller. Create columns of colour with your clothes to help elongate your frame.

Evaluate your body shape and do a little research about your shape on the Internet. There are many websites that will assist with these body shapes, helping you find the best fitting clothing, beneficial exercises, and so on.

Today is Your Day!

Part Three:

Let's keep it simple. If you eat *less* and exercise *more*, you will lose weight. For women, you will eat five times per day every four hours. Men can add a meal if needed; therefore, men can eat up to six times per day. You should lose an average of one to two pounds per week. Exercise will help you lose even more pounds, while keeping your heart healthy. You can do aerobic exercises, jog, skate, play basketball, yoga, play tennis, dance, walk the malls, walk in your neighborhood, swim, cycle, lift weights, march in place, and so on. Do whatever suits your fancy, and you're more likely to make it part of your routine. Just get active. Seek your physician's help to determine your best aerobic heart rate.

As you follow our eating plan for thirty-one days, you will repeat to yourself positive mottos several times each day. In order to begin to heal what has caused you to gain weight, you must change your attitude from the inside out. You will feel good about yourself, as if you were a trophy, a prized possession. But, you cannot be a complete trophy if you just look fit and trim and beautiful or handsome on the outside. You should want to feel great on the inside too. It's eternal.

Dah, it's all about the attitude sometimes!

Part Four:

Allow the thirty-one day regimen schedule to be your daily guide.

1. Follow the Meal Plan
2. Record what you eat throughout the day
3. Recite the daily motto throughout the day
4. Grin, chuckle, and/or laugh as often as you can. Try to *smile* at least twice daily at someone. Watch what happens: it's contagious!

Be mindful of the following:

- Repeat the thirty-one day regimen as many times as needed to lose all the desired weight you want.

- Begin the thirty-one day regimen on the following date of the month you purchased the book. For example, if you purchased this book on October 4, you'd begin the thirty-one day regimen with day 5.

- Smile and have fun. This is your time. The best days of your life awaits you!

Peaches secret weapon to weight-loss:

Squeeze and entire lemon in eight oz of
warm water daily before breakfast.

Day 1

Breakfast:
1 cup of your favorite cereal
2 fruits (i.e. apple, banana, peach, grapes, etc,)
½ cup of milk, (soy, coconut, goat, any dairy, etc.)
At least 8 oz. of water

Snack:
Any 2 oz snack of choice

Lunch:
1 child size hamburger, plain
10 French fries
1 side salad of green veggies (1 cup) with light dressing
6 oz. of soda, juice, or tea
At least 8 oz. of water

Snack:
½ cup of nuts, any kind

Dinner:
6 oz. of lean chicken, baked or grilled
2 cups of cooked fresh veggies, any kind
1 cup of green salad with light dressing
6 oz. of soda, juice, or tea
At least 8 oz. of water

Today's motto:

Don't be afraid, trust yourself. Tell yourself, "I can do this"; "I will do this for me". I will encourage those around me to strive for greater heights. I will not be selfish.

Notes: Jot down what is on your mind.

_____

_____

_____

_____

_____

_____

_____

_____

Day 2

Breakfast:
Breakfast taco, make your own
2 fruits, any (½ cup each)
½ cup of juice, any kind
1 cup of coffee, any style
At least 8 oz. of water

Snack:
Any 2 oz snack of choice

Lunch:
Taco Salad, make your own
6 oz. of soda, juice, or tea
At least 8 oz. of water

Snack:
½ cup of nuts, any kind

Dinner:
6 oz. of lean beef, baked or grilled
2 cups of cooked fresh veggies, any
1 cup of green salad with salsa
6 oz. of soda, juice, or tea
At least 8 oz. of water

Today's motto:

I will be honest. I will treat others like I want to be treated. I will listen to those around me and try to accommodate them to make them smile.

Notes: What happened today?

_____

_____

_____

_____

_____

_____

_____

Day 3

Breakfast:
6 oz of yogurt, any kind
2 fruits, any (½ cup each)
½ cup of juice, any kind
At least 8 oz. of water

Snack:
Any 1 oz snack of choice

Lunch:
6 oz of fish
2 cups of cooked veggies, any kind
6 oz. of soda, juice, or tea
At least 8 oz. of water

Snack:
6 oz of ice cream, any kind

Dinner:
6 oz. of fish, baked or grilled
2 cups of cooked fresh veggies, any
1 cup of green salad with salsa
6 oz. of soda, juice, or tea
At least 8 oz. of water

Today's motto:

I will be quiet and mediate on my inner thoughts. I will not be idle. I will do a good deed to someone that wasn't expecting it.

Notes: Share your feelings.

_____

_____

_____

_____

_____

_____

_____

_____

Day 4

Breakfast:
1 breakfast taco, any kind
2 fruits, any (½ cup each)
½ cup of juice, any kind
1 cup of coffee, any style
At least 8 oz. of water

Snack:
Any 1 oz snack of choice

Lunch:
Chicken sandwich, prepared any style
1 cup of raw veggies, any kind
14 potato chips, any kind
6 oz. of soda, juice, or tea
At least 8 oz. of water

Snack:
¼ cup of bite size candy (i.e. Skittles, M&Ms, etc., any kind)

Dinner:
8 oz. of chicken, baked or grilled
1 small baked potato
1 cup of green salad with salsa
6 oz. of soda, juice, or tea
At least 8 oz. of water

Today's motto:

Be content and at peace with your surroundings. You are approved to live a great life. I will assist in building the strengths of those around me by assisting them with an assignment, objective, or job duty.

Notes: What makes you happy?

_____

_____

_____

_____

_____

_____

_____

Day 5

Breakfast:
1 breakfast omelet, any style
½ cup of hash browns
1 fruits, any kind
½ cup of juice, any kind
At least 8 oz. of water

Snack:
½ cup of applesauce or jello

Lunch:
Any sandwich, prepared any style
2 cup of raw veggies, any kind
6 oz. of soda, juice, or tea
At least 8 oz. of water

Snack:
½ cup of nuts, any kind

Dinner:
8 oz. of veal or beef, baked or grilled
½ cup of pasta, any style
2 cups of green salad with salsa
6 oz. of soda, juice, or tea
At least 8 oz. of water

Today's motto:

I will have a teachable and diplomatic attitude today. I will give those around me their personal space and be unswerving.

Notes: What makes you excited?

_____

_____

_____

_____

_____

_____

_____

Day 6

Breakfast:
1 biscuit
2 tsp of jelly, jam, or preserve
1 oz. of meat or protein substitute
2 fruits, any (½ cup each)
½ cup of juice, any kind
1 cup of coffee, any style
At least 8 oz. of water

Snack:
Any 2 oz snack of choice

Lunch:
Taco Salad with 2 cups of green salad
7 tortilla chips
½ cup of salsa
6 oz. of soda, juice, or tea
At least 8 oz. of water

Snack:
½ cup of nuts, any kind

Dinner:
8 oz. of fish, baked or grilled
½ cup of rice pilaf
2 cups of green salad with salsa
6 oz. of soda, juice, or tea
At least 8 oz. of water

Today's motto:

I will not worry about anything anymore. I will look to the future with great anticipation of the unknown. I will show love around my family and friends like I've never done before.

Notes: What makes you less happy or sad?

_____

_____

_____

_____

_____

_____

_____

Day 7

Breakfast:
~Your choice~

Snack:
1 serving of pudding

Lunch:
3 oz. of meat, any style
1 small baked potato, made any style
2 veggies (1/2 cup each)
8 oz. of soda, juice, or tea
At least 8 oz. of water

Dinner:
1 bowl of soup, any kind
2 cup of green salad with salsa
6 oz. of soda, juice, or tea
At least 8 oz. of water

Dessert:
2 oz of your desired preference

Today's motto:

I am awesome. I got this! I will be courteous and civil to all those who cross my path today.

Notes: What is happiness to you?

_____

_____

_____

_____

_____

_____

_____

_____

Day 8

Breakfast:
1 cup of your favorite cereal
2 fruits, any (½ cup each)
½ cup of milk, (soy, coconut, goat, any dairy, etc.)
At least 8 oz. of water

Snack:
Any 1 oz snack of choice

Lunch:
1 medium size cheeseburger,
7 French fries
1 side salad of green veggies (1 cup) with light dressing
6 oz. of soda, juice, or tea
At least 8 oz. of water

Snack:
6 oz of cottage cheese with fruit, any kind

Dinner:
7 oz. of lean chicken, baked or grilled
2 cups of fresh veggies, any
1 cup of green salad with light dressing
6 oz. of soda, juice, or tea
At least 8 oz. of water

Today's motto:

I will be patient with my progress. I will not grumble or be irritated to those around me.

Notes: Jot you're your innermost thoughts.

_____

_____

_____

_____

_____

_____

_____

Day 9

Breakfast:
2 egg or protein substitute
1 oz of breakfast meat, any kind
2 fruits, any (½ cup each)
½ cup of juice, any kind
1 cup of coffee, any style
At least 8 oz. of water

Snack:
Any 2 oz snack of choice

Lunch:
1 seafood or Caesar Salad, with light dressing
1 cup of raw veggies
6 oz. of soda, juice, or tea
At least 8 oz. of water

Snack:
½ cup of nuts, any kind

Dinner:
8 oz. of lean chicken, baked or grilled
2 cups of cooked fresh veggies, any
1 cup of green salad with light dressing
6 oz. of soda, juice, or tea
At least 8 oz. of water

Today's motto:

I will begin writing down my goals for the next 3 years. I will encourage others to do the same. I will not be judgmental if they do not respond.

Notes: Share your thoughts today.

_____

_____

_____

_____

_____

_____

_____

_____

Day 10

Breakfast:
8 oz of yogurt, any kind
2 fruits, any (½ cup each)
½ cup of juice, any kind
At least 8 oz. of water

Snack:
Any 1 oz snack of choice

Lunch:
8 oz of fish
1 cup of cooked veggies, any kind
10 oz. of soda, juice, or tea
At least 8 oz. of water

Snack:
½ cup of ice cream, any kind

Dinner:
8 oz. of pork or other protein, baked or grilled
2 cups of fresh veggies, any
1 cup of green salad with light dressing
8 oz. of soda, juice, or tea
At least 8 oz. of water

Today's motto:

I will review what has been bothering me. I will confront the problem. If I've made wrong choices, I will forgive myself and do better. If others have said negative things to me or wronged me, I will continue to be nice and not hold grudges against them.

Notes: What's the problem?

_____

_____

_____

_____

_____

_____

_____

Day 11

Breakfast:
1 breakfast taco, any kind
2 fruits, any (½ cup each)
½ cup of juice, any kind
1 cup of coffee, any style
At least 8 oz. of water

Snack:
Any 2 oz snack of choice

Lunch:
Roast beef sandwich, prepared any style
1 cup of raw veggies, any kind
10 potato chips, any kind
8 oz. of soda, juice, or tea
At least 8 oz. of water

Snack:
½ cup of nuts, any kind

Dinner:
8 oz. of fish, baked or grilled
1 small baked potato
1 cup of green salad with light dressing
8 oz. of soda, juice, or tea
At least 8 oz. of water

Today's motto:

I will read my favorite book. I will blog about my favorite book. If someone confides in me, I will not judge. I will be trustworthy and true.

Notes: Did you read today?

_____

_____

_____

_____

_____

_____

_____

_____

Day 12

Breakfast:
1 breakfast omelet, any style
½ cup of hash browns
1 fruits, any kind
½ cup of juice, any kind
At least 8 oz. of water

Snack:
Any 1 oz snack of choice

Lunch:
1 personal pizza, prepared any style
2 cup of raw veggies, any kind
8 oz. of soda, juice, or tea
At least 8 oz. of water

Snack:
6 oz of yogurt, any kind

Dinner:
8 oz. of Lasagna, any style
½ cup of pasta, any style
2 cup of green salad with light dressing
6 oz. of soda, juice, or tea
At least 8 oz. of water

Today's motto:

I will not be discouraged today even though a situation did not go in my favor. I will complete all my commitments to my friends and family.

Notes: Did you complete your to-do list today?

_____

_____

_____

_____

_____

_____

_____

_____

Day 13

Breakfast:
2 small waffles
2 tsp of jelly, jam, or syrup
2 oz. of meat or protein substitute
2 fruits, any (½ cup each)
½ cup of juice, any kind
1 cup of coffee, any style
At least 8 oz. of water

Snack:
Any 2 oz snack of choice

Lunch:
Tuna Salad with 2 cups of green salad
32 small corn chips
8 oz. of soda, juice, or tea
At least 8 oz. of water

Snack:
Men only: ½ cup of nuts, any kind

Dinner:
8 oz. of beef, baked or grilled
½ cup of rice pilaf
2 cup of green salad with light dressing
8 oz. of soda, juice, or tea
At least 8 oz. of water

Today's motto:
I will smile until it hurts me. I will laugh more. I will love life. I will make all promises to family and friends come into fruition.

Notes: How many times did you smile today, and why?

_____

_____

_____

_____

_____

_____

_____

Day 14

Breakfast:
~Your choice~

Snack:
1 serving of favorite snack

Lunch:
8 oz. of meat, any style
1 cup of soup, any style
2 veggies (1/2 cup each)
8 oz. of soda, juice, or tea
At least 8 oz. of water

Dinner:
4 oz. of protein
2 cup of green salad with light dressing
6 oz. of soda, juice, or tea
At least 8 oz. of water

Dessert:
2 oz of your desired preference

Today's motto:

I can do anything I put mind to do. I am the best me I can be. I will not give up on friends, co-workers, or family, no matter how much they annoy me.

Notes: What makes you strive to be the best you today? If not, why?

_____

_____

_____

_____

_____

_____

_____

_____

The next 15 days will feature meals from the "EAT THIS NOT THAT" book by David Zinczenko with Matt Goulding, Rodal Inc. (2010)

Day 15

Breakfast:
1 cup of your favorite cereal
2 fruits, any (½ cup each)
½ cup of milk, (soy, coconut, goat, any dairy, etc.)
At least 8 oz. of water

Snack:
6 oz of applesauce

Lunch:
1 small personal pizza, any style *(or a Grilled Dijon Chicken from Applebee's)*
1 side salad of green veggies (1 cup) with salsa
6 oz. of soda, juice, or tea
At least 8 oz. of water

Snack:
½ cup of nuts, any kind

Dinner:
7 oz. of lean chicken, baked or grilled
2 cups of fresh veggies, any
1 cup of green salad with salsa
6 oz. of soda, juice, or tea
At least 8 oz. of water

Today's motto:

I will stay modest with my success. I will encourage others to try my 31 Day regimen. If they refuse, I will smile and return to what I was doing previously.

Notes: Did you encourage someone today? If so, who and why?

_____

_____

_____

_____

_____

_____

_____

_____

Day 16

Breakfast:
2 egg or protein substitute
1 oz of breakfast meat, any kind
2 fruits, any (½ cup each)
½ cup of juice, any kind
1 cup of coffee, any style
At least 8 oz. of water

Snack:
Any 2 oz snack of choice

Lunch:
1 Chef Salad, with light dressing *(or a Chicken Torta from Baja Fresh)*
1 cup of cooked veggies
8 oz. of soda, juice, or tea
At least 8 oz. of water

Snack:
½ cup of nuts, any kind

Dinner:
8 oz. of lean chicken, baked or grilled
2 cups of cooked fresh veggies, any
1 cup of green salad with salsa
6 oz. of soda, juice, or tea
At least 8 oz. of water

Today's motto:

I will write in a journal about the first 16 days of this 31 Day regimen. I will be my friends and family cheerleader to their dreams and/or goals.

Notes: Jot down what you are feeling at this very moment in time.

_____

_____

_____

_____

_____

_____

_____

_____

Day 17

Breakfast:
8 oz of yogurt, any kind
2 fruits, any (½ cup each)
½ cup of juice, any kind
At least 8 oz. of water

Snack:
Any 2 oz snack or chips

Lunch:
8 oz of fish
1 cup of cooked veggies, any kind
10 oz. of soda, juice, or tea
At least 8 oz. of water

Snack:
¼ cup of candy bites, any kind

Dinner:
8 oz. of pork or other protein, baked or grilled (*or homemade grilled Chicken tacos*)
2 cups of fresh veggies, any
1 cup of green salad with salsa
8 oz. of soda, juice, or tea
At least 8 oz. of water

Today's motto:

I will not fear any problem, person, or predicament. I choose to look to the future for the answer. I will buy an individual's lunch today.

Notes: What are your fears? How long have they been fears?

_____

_____

_____

_____

_____

_____

_____

_____

Day 18

Breakfast:
1 breakfast taco, any kind
2 fruits, any (½ cup each)
½ cup of juice, any kind
1 cup of coffee, any style
At least 8 oz. of water

Snack:
Any 1 oz snack of choice

Lunch:
Cold cut sandwich, prepared any style
1 cup of raw veggies, any kind
10 potato chips, any kind
8 oz. of soda, juice, or tea
At least 8 oz. of water

Snack:
½ cup of pudding, any kind

Dinner:
8 oz. of fish, baked or grilled *(or a Margarita Grilled Chicken entrée from Chili's)*
1 small baked potato
1 cup of green salad with salsa
8 oz. of soda, juice, or tea
At least 8 oz. of water

Today's motto:

I will find time to relax and rest. I will donate some unutilized items in my home or office to an organization or charity. I will commit to volunteering at a shelter at least one hour per 6 months.

Notes: Did you rest today? What did you have to do to take time out for yourself?

_____

_____

_____

_____

_____

_____

_____

_____

Day 19

Breakfast:
1 breakfast omelet, any style
½ cup of hash browns
1 fruits, any kind
½ cup of juice, any kind
At least 8 oz. of water

Snack:
Any 2 oz snack of choice

Lunch:
6 oz. of Asian style meat
1 cup of Fried rice
1 cup of cooked veggies, any kind
8 oz. of soda, juice, or tea
At least 8 oz. of water

Snack:
½ cup of nuts, any kind

Dinner:
8 oz. of Lasagna, any style *(or a Steak Burrito Bowl from Chipotle)*
½ cup of pasta, any style
2 cup of green salad with light dressing
6 oz. of soda, juice, or tea
At least 8 oz. of water

Today's motto:
I will love myself, my family, and my friends no matter what.

Notes: Do you love You? Jot down 3 things you like about yourself and why.

_____

_____

_____

_____

_____

_____

_____

_____

Day 20

Breakfast:
2 small pancakes *(or two egg & cheese wake-up wraps from Dunkin' Donuts)*
2 tsp of jelly, jam, or syrup
2 oz. of meat or protein substitute
2 fruits, any (½ cup each)
½ cup of juice, any kind
1 cup of coffee, any style
At least 8 oz. of water

Snack:
Any 2 oz snack of choice

Lunch:
Chicken Salad with 2 cups of green salad
2 fruits, any kind
8 oz. of soda, juice, or tea
At least 8 oz. of water

Snack:
½ cup of nuts, any kind

Dinner:
8 oz. of beef, baked or grilled
½ cup of rice pilaf
2 cup of green salad with salsa
8 oz. of soda, juice, or tea
At least 8 oz. of water

Today's motto:

I choose to live a satisfied life without complaining. I will be positive to those around me even when they are not.

Notes: What did you complain about today and why did it bother you?

_____

_____

_____

_____

_____

_____

_____

_____

Day 21
(Half Day Fast – no food only liquids)

Breakfast:
12oz of protein shake any kind

Lunch:
1 bowl of broth

Dinner:
4 oz. of protein
2 cup of green salad with salsa
6 oz. of soda, juice, or tea
At least 8 oz. of water

Dessert:
2 oz of your desired preference

Today's motto:

I will be thankful for my life. I will attend a self-help seminar to improve my personal or business skills within 7 months of reading this book.

Notes: What are 2 items about yourself that you are working on improving?

_____

_____

_____

_____

_____

_____

_____

_____

Day 22

Breakfast:
1 cup of your favorite cereal
2 fruits, any (½ cup each)
½ cup of milk, (soy, coconut, goat, any dairy, etc.)
At least 8 oz. of water

Snack:
Any 2 oz snack of choice

Lunch:
1 child size hamburger, plain *(or two fresco Crunchy tacos and Pintos 'n Cheese from Taco Bell)*
10 French fries
1 side salad of green veggies (1 cup) with light dressing
6 oz. of soda, juice, or tea
At least 8 oz. of water

Snack:
½ cup of jello, any kind

Dinner:
6 oz. of lean chicken, baked or grilled
2 cups of cooked fresh veggies, any
1 cup of green salad with light dressing
6 oz. of soda, juice, or tea
At least 8 oz. of water

Today's motto:

Don't be afraid, remember the challenging times. You overcame them. Encourage others to do the same. Lead by being an example.

Notes: Name 1 challenging you are dealing with and why.

_____

_____

_____

_____

_____

_____

_____

Day 23

Breakfast:
1 egg or protein substitute
1 oz of breakfast meat, any kind
2 fruits, any (½ cup each)
½ cup of juice, any kind
1 cup of coffee, any style
At least 8 oz. of water

Snack:
Any 1 oz snack of choice

Lunch:
1 Chef Salad, 2 cups of mixed greens with salsa
1 cup of raw veggies
6 oz. of soda, juice, or tea
At least 8 oz. of water

Snack:
½ cup of nuts, any kind

Dinner:
6 oz. of lean beef, baked or grilled (or a Flat Iron Steak entrée from T.G.I. Friday's)
2 cups of cooked fresh veggies, any
1 cup of green salad with salsa
6 oz. of soda, juice, or tea
At least 8 oz. of water

Today's motto:

I will keep my mind and my imagination on ideas that are pleasant and pleasing. I will recognize any roots or resentment and yield that resentment to being optimistic.

Notes: What pleases you the most?

_____

_____

_____

_____

_____

_____

_____

_____

Day 24

Breakfast:
6 oz of yogurt, any kind
2 fruits, any (½ cup each)
½ cup of juice, any kind
At least 8 oz. of water

Snack:
8 oz smoothie, any kind

Lunch:
6 oz of fish
2 cups of cooked veggies, any kind
6 oz. of soda, juice, or tea
At least 8 oz. of water

Snack:
1 oz of baked chips, any kind

Dinner:
6 oz. of fish, baked or grilled *(or homemade meat Lasagna or from Sbarro)*
2 cups of cooked fresh veggies, any
1 cup of green salad with salsa
6 oz. of soda, juice, or tea
At least 8 oz. of water

Today's motto:

I will be trustworthy and operate my daily activities in integrity. I will be fair and considerate to those around me.

Notes: Are you trustworthy? What are you doing to keep character in check?

_____

_____

_____

_____

_____

_____

_____

_____

Day 25

Breakfast:
1 breakfast taco, any kind
2 fruits, any (½ cup each)
½ cup of juice, any kind
1 cup of coffee, any style
At least 8 oz. of water

Snack:
Any 2 oz snack of choice

Lunch:
Chicken sandwich, prepared any style
1 cup of raw veggies, any kind
14 potato chips, any kind
6 oz. of soda, juice, or tea
At least 8 oz. of water

Snack:
½ cup of nuts, any kind

Dinner:
8 oz. of chicken, grilled *(or Peach-Bourbon BBQ Shrimp and Scallops from Red Lobster)*
1 small baked potato
1 cup of green salad with light dressing
6 oz. of soda, juice, or tea
At least 8 oz. of water

Today's motto:

I have many problems; but, I will work through them till they are no longer problems. I will live a balanced life. I will work and volunteer in my community to make it a better place.

Notes: What are small problems? What makes them problems?

_____

_____

_____

_____

_____

_____

_____

Day 26

Breakfast:
1 breakfast omelet, any style
½ cup of hash browns
1 fruits, any kind
½ cup of juice, any kind
At least 8 oz. of water

Snack:
Any 1 oz snack of choice

Lunch:
Any sandwich, prepared any style
2 cup of raw veggies, any kind
6 oz. of soda, juice, or tea
At least 8 oz. of water

Snack:
½ cup of nuts, any kind

Dinner:
8 oz. of veal or beef, baked or grilled *(or Asian Marinated NY Strip Steak from P.F. Chang's)*
½ cup of pasta, any style
2 cups of green salad with salsa
6 oz. of soda, juice, or tea
At least 8 oz. of water

Today's motto:
I will fight for justice. I will not be unfair despite my political views. I will protect my family and those I love.

Notes: What does justice mean to me?

_____

_____

_____

_____

_____

_____

_____

Day 27

Breakfast:
1 biscuit
2 tsp of jelly, jam, or preserve
1 oz. of meat or protein substitute
2 fruits, any (½ cup each)
½ cup of juice, any kind
1 cup of coffee, any style
At least 8 oz. of water

Snack:
Any 2 oz snack of choice

Lunch:
Taco Salad made your way *(or a bowl of Tortilla soup from Boston Market or homemade)*
7 tortilla chips
½ cup of salsa
6 oz. of soda, juice, or tea
At least 8 oz. of water

Snack:
½ cup of nuts, any kind

Dinner:
8 oz. of fish, baked or grilled
½ cup of rice pilaf
2 cups of green salad with salsa
6 oz. of soda, juice, or tea
At least 8 oz. of water

Today's motto:

I will laugh at least 3 times today for 15 seconds. I will smile more. I will assist those around me to complete their desired dreams and/ or goals. I will offer my support if they need it.

Notes: Did you laugh today? Describe what happened.

_____

_____

_____

_____

_____

_____

_____

_____

Day 28

Breakfast:
~Your choice~

Snack:
1 serving of pudding

Lunch:
6 oz. of meat, any style
1 small baked potato, made any style
2 veggies (1/2 cup each)
8 oz. of soda, juice, or tea
At least 8 oz. of water

Dinner:
1 bowl of soup, any kind
2 cup of green salad with salsa
6 oz. of soda, juice, or tea
At least 8 oz. of water

Dessert:
2 oz of your desired preference

Today's motto:

Let there be light in my day. I will appreciate the beautiful sunrise and sunset today. I will offer a helping hand to someone in need.

Notes: Name 3 things that you thought were beautiful today?

_____

_____

_____

_____

_____

_____

_____

Day 29

Breakfast:
2 small waffles
2 tsp of jelly, jam, or syrup
2 oz. of meat or protein substitute
2 fruits, any (½ cup each)
½ cup of juice, any kind
1 cup of coffee, any style
At least 8 oz. of water

Snack:
Any 2 oz snack of choice

Lunch:
Tuna Salad with 2 cups of green salad
32 small corn chips
8 oz. of soda, juice, or tea
At least 8 oz. of water

Snack:
½ cup of nuts, any kind

Dinner:
8 oz. of beef, baked or grilled *(or chicken fajitas with onions from On the Border or homemade)*
½ cup of rice pilaf
2 cup of green salad with salsa
8 oz. of soda, juice, or tea
At least 8 oz. of water

Today's motto:

I will trust my instincts regarding my future and my happiness. I will no longer give way to those negative thoughts that was holding me hostage. I have a new life that is filled with love, joy, and peace. I will spread that joy to others through my actions and reactions.

Notes: What does trust mean to you? Are you considered a negative person? What makes you that way and/or the opposite - happy?

_____

_____

_____

_____

_____

_____

_____

_____

Day 30

Breakfast:
~Your choice~

Snack:
Men and Women: 1 serving of favorite snack

Lunch:
8 oz. of meat, any style
1 cup of soup, any style
2 veggies (1/2 cup each)
8 oz. of soda, juice, or tea
At least 8 oz. of water

Dinner:
4 oz. of protein
2 cup of green salad with light dressing
6 oz. of soda, juice, or tea
At least 8 oz. of water

Dessert:
2 oz of your desired preference

Today's motto:

I will hold on to what I have learned through this 31 Day regimen. I can conquer any adversity with a positive attitude. I will serve others with pure motives.

Notes: What makes you dedicated to losing weight?

_____

_____

_____

_____

_____

_____

_____

_____

Day 31

Create your own plan. You can do it!

If you have less than ten pounds to lose, below is Peaches quick start regimen. Follow the plan for seven days only:
   Breakfast – any meal totaling 350 calories
   Lunch – any meal totaling 1,050 calories
   Dinner – 8 oz of chicken or beef broth

Drink water, green tea, or black coffee with all meals. No diet drinks. No snacks or eating between meals.
Recite Psalms 121 daily for 7 days

The LORD Is Thy Keeper, *Psalms 121*

1 I will lift up mine eyes unto the hills,
   from whence cometh my help.
2 My help *cometh* from the LORD,
   which made heaven and earth.
3 He will not suffer thy foot to be moved:
   he that keepeth thee will not slumber.
4 Behold, he that keepeth Israel
   shall neither slumber nor sleep.
5 The LORD *is* thy keeper:
   the LORD *is* thy shade upon thy right hand.
6 The sun shall not smite thee by day,
   nor the moon by night.
7 The LORD shall preserve thee from all evil:
   he shall preserve thy soul.
8 The LORD shall preserve thy going out and thy coming in
   from this time forth, and even for evermore.

Recipes:

Southern Grilled Chicken Breast

Ingredients:

- o ¼ cup of onion power
- o ¼ cup of paprika
- o 1 ½ tbsps of chili powder
- o ½ tsp of Accent flavor enhancer
- o ¼ tsp of red pepper
- o ½ cup of lemon juice
- o 1 tbsp of garlic power
- o 1 ½ tsps of salt
- o 5 chicken breasts

Mix all the dry ingredients together. Pour in a plastic bag. Place the chicken breasts in the bag and shake. Marinate in the refrigerator for almost 2 hours. Grill the chicken for about 18 minutes turning occasionally or until done.

Southern Grilled Fish
(Tilapia, Flounder, Catfish, or whatever type of fish you like)

Ingredients:

- o ¼ cup Cajun Seasoning
- o ¼ tsp of paprika
- o ½ cup of browning flavoring sauce
- o ½ tsp of Accent flavor enhancer
- o ¼ tsp of red pepper
- o ½ tsp of salt
- o 5 fish fillets

Mix all the dry ingredients together. Pour in a plastic bag. Place the fillets in the bag and shake. Pour the browning sauce evenly on the fish. Marinate in the refrigerator for 30 minutes. Grill the fish for about 7 minutes turning a couple of times or until done.

Kiss yo Momma Chicken & Rice Soup

Ingredients:

- ¼ cup of onion power or 1 whole white onion
- ¼ cup of garlic power or 3 cloves of garlic
- 7 cups of chicken broth
- 1 tbsp of Accent flavor enhancer
- ¼ tsp of red pepper
- ½ cup of finely cut celery
- ¼ cup of bell pepper
- 1 cup of fresh carrots
- 1 cup of fresh mushrooms
- 1 stick of butter or margarine
- ½ cup of flour
- 1 ¾ cup of rice (white, brown, or wild)
- 1 ½ tsps of salt
- Dash of curry powder
- 1 ½ cups of cream (half & half)
- 5 chicken breasts

Sauté the onion, garlic, celery, bell pepper, and carrots in butter for 7 minutes, then add the mushrooms. Cook for 3 minutes. Add the flour evenly and cook for 3 minutes. Add the chicken broth and boil for 1 minute. Reduce heat and add the rice, salt, curry powder, Accent flavor enhancer, and red pepper. Simmer for 7 minutes before adding the cream. Continue to simmer for about an hour or until the taste pleases your palate.

Jamaican-American Jerk Pork

Ingredients:

- o ¼ cup of onion power
- o ½ cup of Jamaican Jerk seasoning
- o 1 ½ tbsps of cumin
- o ½ tsp of Accent flavor enhancer
- o ¼ tsp of red pepper
- o ½ cup of lime juice
- o 1 tbsp of garlic power
- o 1 ½ tsps of salt
- o 2 lbs of Pork tenderloins

Mix all the dry ingredients together. Pour in a plastic bag. Place the pork tenderloins in the bag and shake. Spread the Jamaican Jerk seasoning on the pork tenderloins and place in the refrigerator for almost 1 hour. Cook the pork turning occasionally or until done.

TexMex Lasagna

Ingredients:

- 3 tbsps of vegetable oil
- 2 lbs of ground sirloin
- 3 tbsps of chili powder
- ½ cup of chopped green onion (scallions)
- 1 tsp of Accent flavor enhancer
- 1 tsp of red pepper
- 3 tsps of cumin
- 1 (8 oz) can of beans (ranch style, kidney, black), drained
- 1 tbsp of garlic power
- 1 (16 oz) can of Mexican stewed tomatoes
- 1 cup of corn
- 1 ½ tsps of salt
- 7 lite-carb tortillas,
- 1 cup of shredded Cheddar cheese
- 2 cups of mozzarella cheese

Cook ground sirloin in vegetable oil using all the dry seasonings. Once meat is brown, add the stewed tomatoes, beans, and corn. Cook for 3 minutes and add salt.

Preheat oven to 450 degrees F. Coat the baking pan with vegetable oil. Layer the meat and beans mixture, mozzarella cheese, and tortillas to your satisfaction. Repeat the layers until all the ingredients are used. Bake the Lasagna for 16 minutes until cheese is brown. Top with green onion and shredded cheddar cheese and enjoy.

Texas Fried Chicken

Ingredients:

- o   1 tbsp of onion power
- o   2 eggs
- o   ¼ cup of TexJoy steak seasoning
- o   ½ tsp of Accent flavor enhancer
- o   ¼ tsp of red pepper
- o   1 tbsp of garlic power
- o   1 ½ tsps ob salt
- o   1 1/2 cups of flour
- o   1 ½ lbs of chicken
- o   Vegetable oil, for frying

Heat the oil around 370 degrees in a large pot. Place the flour aside. Mix all the dry ingredients together. Pour in a plastic bag. Place the chicken in the bag and shake. Beat the eggs and set aside. Dip the seasoned chicken in the egg, and then coat well in the flour. Put the chicken in the oil and fry until brown and crisp turning occasionally. Cooking time is approximately 16-18 minutes.

TexMex Roast Beef

Ingredients:

- o   1 tbsp of onion power
- o   1 tsp of celery power
- o   2 tbsps of chili powder
- o   1 tsp of Accent flavor enhancer
- o   1 tsp of red pepper
- o   1tbsp of cumin
- o   1 tbsp of garlic power
- o   1 ½ tsps of salt
- o   3 lbs of beef brisket
- o   2 cups of beef broth
- o   1 ½ tsps of dry mustard

Preheat oven to 325 degrees F. Mix all the dry ingredients together. Rub on beef. Place in roasting pan for 2 hours. Add beef broth and cook covered for 2 hours, or until tender

Summer Day Chicken Salad

Ingredients:

- o   1 tsp of onion power
- o   1 tbsp of chopped green onion (scallions)
- o   2 tbsp of chopped white onion
- o   2 tbsp of chopped celery
- o   2 boiled eggs, chopped
- o   2 tbsps of pickle relish
- o   ½ cup of mayonnaise or salad dressing
- o   ½ tsp of Accent flavor enhancer
- o   ¼ tsp of red pepper
- o   ½ tsp of salt
- o   1 lb of chicken

Combine all ingredients in a large bowl and enjoy.

TexMex Lamb Chops

Ingredients:

- o 1 tbsp of onion power
- o 1 tsp of celery power
- o 2 tbsps of chili powder
- o 1 tsp of Accent flavor enhancer
- o 1 tsp of red pepper
- o 1 tbsp of cumin
- o 1 tbsp of garlic power
- o 1 ½ tsps of salt
- o 3 lbs of lamb chops

Preheat oven to 325 degrees F. Mix all the dry ingredients together. Rub on lamb chops. Place in roasting pan or cast iron skillet for 1 hour or until tender. Let cool and enjoy!

Texan Veal Chops

Ingredients:

- o   1 tbsp of onion power
- o   1 tbsp of celery power
- o   2 bay leaves
- o   1 tsp of Accent flavor enhancer
- o   1 tsp of red pepper
- o   1tbsp of cumin
- o   1 tbsp of garlic power
- o   1 ½ tsps of salt
- o   3 lbs of lamb chops
- o   1 chopped red onion
- o   1 cup of fresh carrots
- o   ¾ cup of chopped celery
- o   1 cup of chicken broth
- o   1/3 cup of butter
- o   Oil for pan

Mix all the dry ingredients together. Rub on veal chops. Sauté in pan over medium heat and cook chops until brown. Set chops aside. Sauté red onion, carrots, celery and bay leaves in oil for about 12 minutes. Add the broth and butter to the vegetables and cook for 7 minutes. Place the chops in the mixture and cook uncovered for 12 minutes and enjoy.

Remember: "Casting all your care upon him; for He careth for you" I Peter 5:7

References:

http://www.buzzle.com/articles/pear-shaped-body-type.html

Mateijan, G. (2006). The world's healthiest foods, *Essential guide for the healthiest way of eating*. 1st Ed. Seattle Washington

Scripture quotations taken from the New King James Version®. Copyright © 1982 by Thomas Nelson, Inc. Used by permission. All rights reserved.

Shamblin, G. (1997). Weigh Down Diet. 1st Ed.,New York, New York. Doubleday Publishers.

www.**cdc.gov/obesity**/data. Retrieved on December 26, 2012.

www.fatfree.com. Retrieved on December 26, 2012.

www.eatright.org. Retrieved on December 26, 2012.

~The End~

About the Author

Peaches Monroe, is a wife, mother, and special educational consultant in Texas. Please send your comments and/or if you need encouragement in any form, please email her at peachesmonroetexmex@yahoo.com. Ms. Monroe and her husband reside in Texas.

www.ingramcontent.com/pod-product-compliance
Lightning Source LLC
Chambersburg PA
CBHW030353290526
45785CB00004B/1732